Dedication

To my wife. Your dedication to our family is second to none. Always a beacon of hope during difficult times.

To my mom. Your bravery and faith has never wavered while you walked through the valley of shadow and death.

You're both an inspiration and great examples of godly women.

I love you both.

Introduction

Who are you?

I'm just someone who's been living with back pain and has learned to maintain a modest lifestyle over the years.

I currently live with Chronic Kidney Disease, on stage 3 as of the writing of this edition.

Everything on this book I've tried myself, know someone who has, or I've done research as to who's tried them.

Where did these recipes come from?

I've done a lot of research and found these from the Internet, people I know, books, etc. I've put the best here so you don't have to spend years looking like I have.

Edition 4 Updates

I added a quick introduction into teas and how they've helped me.

READ THIS DISCLAIMER

I AM NOT A DOCTOR! I made this book by doing research and using these juices on my self. My mom did many of these while she was doing chemo and I attribute her juice fast to her survival, but that is my opinion.

I have no allergies to any fruits and vegetables so if you do, make sure you DO NOT JUICE THAT RECIPE.

Consult with your doctor first! As always, if you're going to start a diet or workout routine with any health issues, please consult with your family doctor.

I legally cannot advocate for the results that the name of these juices may suggest. The opinions found in this book are mine and mine alone. I do not claim that these recipes cure anything.

Finally, the creators of the images throughout this book may not endorse what is said in this book. Their images was used with permission from UnSplash.com. Their credits are at the back of this book.

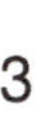

Juices

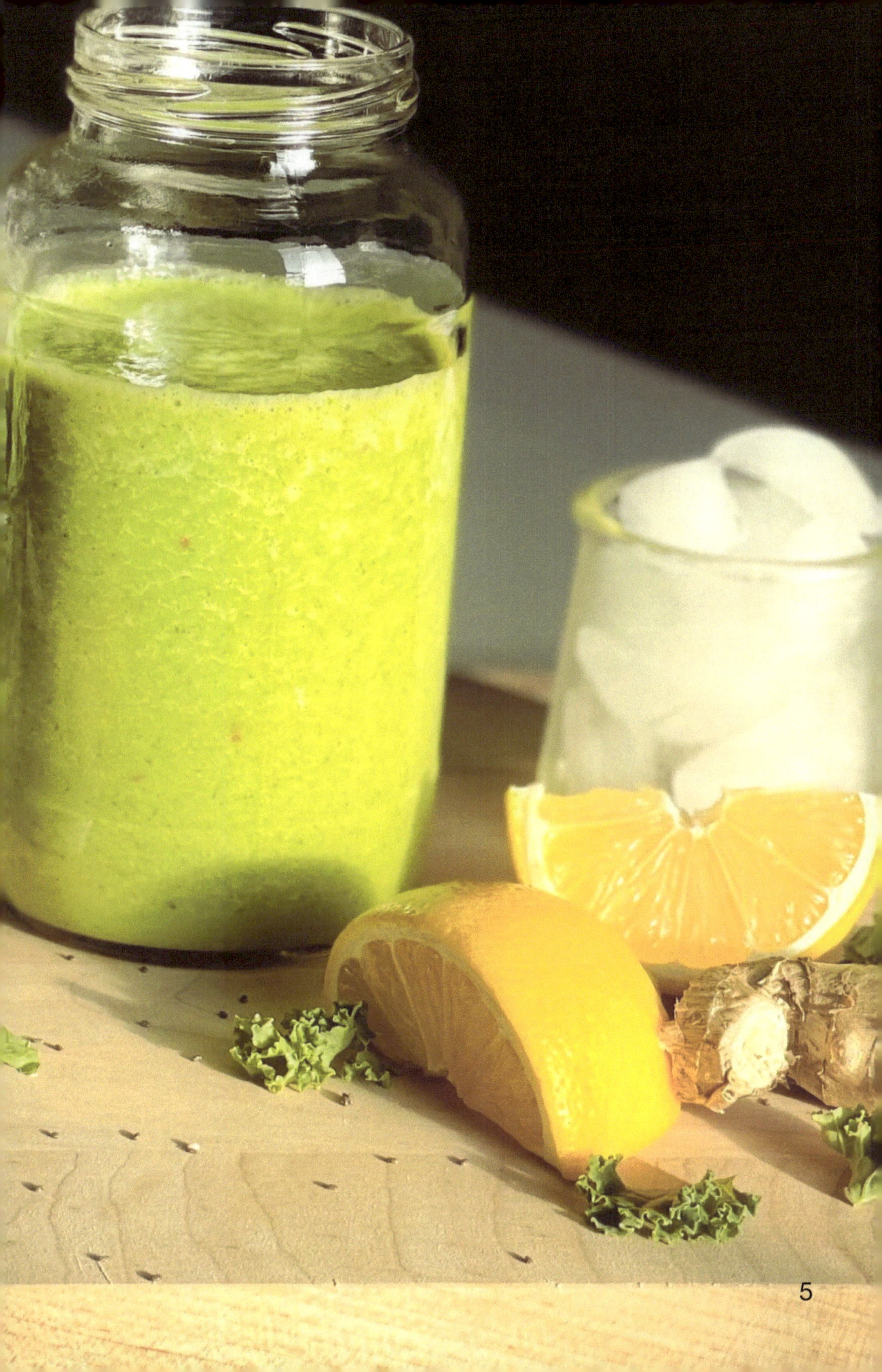

THE MEAN GREEN

This is a very brutal detoxification juice. This will jump start your body but not before you feel the effects years of junk food had on you. Made famous by the Joe Cross documentary, "Fat, Sick, and Nearly Dead". A documentary worth watching.

- ➡ 6 KALE LEAVES
- ➡ 1 CUCUMBER
- ➡ 4 CELERY STALKS
- ➡ 2 GREEN APPLES
- ➡ 1/2 LEMON
- ➡ 1 PIECE OF GINGER

The Light Green

The lightest of the primary meals. This primary meal is for those who have difficulty with the first two.

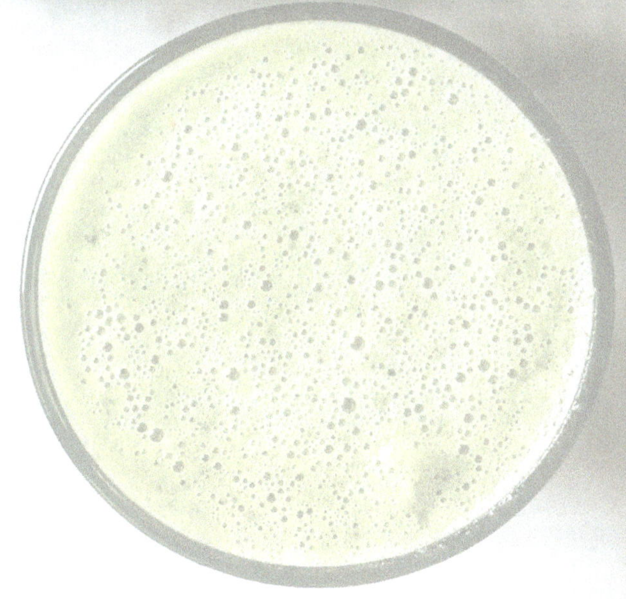

- ➡ 1 BIG HANDFUL OF SPINACH
- ➡ 3 LARGE STALKS CELERY
- ➡ 1/2 ENGLISH CUCUMBER (PEEL ON)
- ➡ 5 CHERRY TOMATOES
- ➡ 1 GARLIC CLOVE
- ➡ 1/4 CUP CARROT JUICE
- ➡ 1/2 CUP FILTERED WATER

My Favorite

I can drink this all the day long! Very very delicious and very nutritious!

➡ 3 Medium or 2 Large Carrots
➡ 1 Apple

If you're wondering what kind of apples to use, choose your favorite! These work best: Granny Smith, Macintosh, Ida Red, Pippin, or Gala

FERTILITY HELPER

The name says it all!

- ➡ 3 HARD PEARS
- ➡ 1 CANTALOUPE
- ➡ 1 SWEET POTATO

Detox Rush

This is a good rush detoxifier. Drink lots of water throughout the day.

- ➡ 1 LEMON
- ➡ 2 RADISH
- ➡ 1 BEET
- ➡ 1 SLICE SPANISH ONION
- ➡ 2 SWEET POTATO
- ➡ 1 CELERY
- ➡ 2 TBS. CIDER VINEGAR

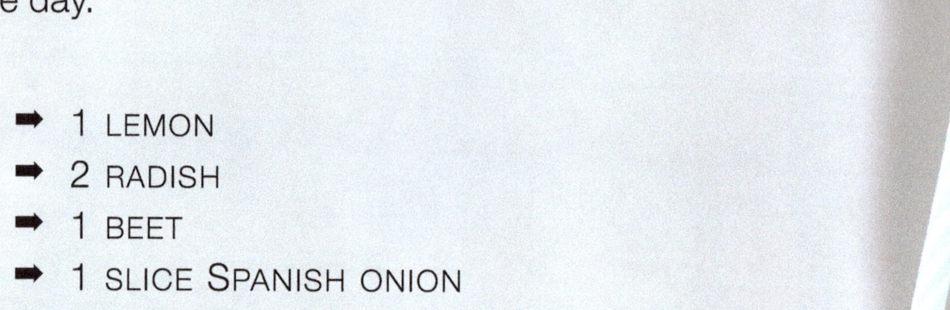

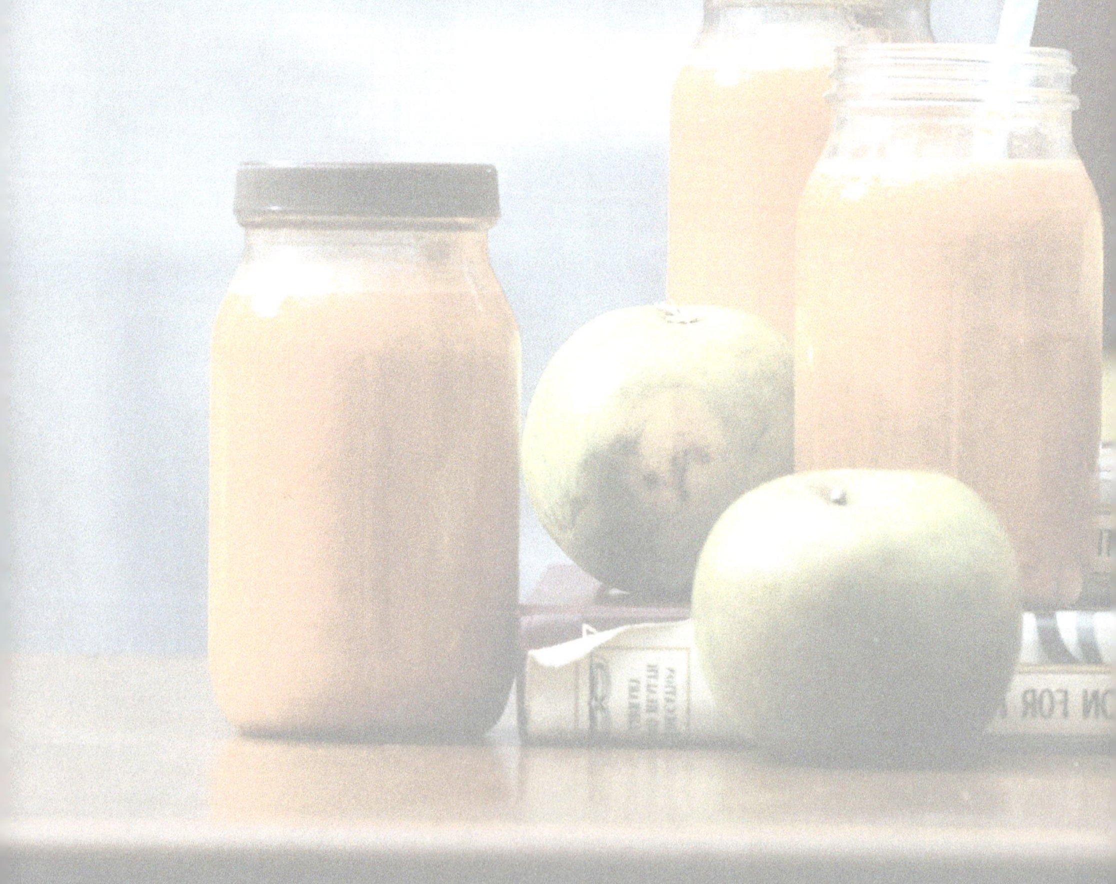

Natural Pain Killer

When you get hurt, things like sprains, bruises, and even normal aches can be aggravated if you have a high protein diet. This juice, in combination with a low protein macro diet (raw fruits and veggies), will help reduce these aggravations. Oh, and it tastes great!

- ➡ 1 LEMON
- ➡ 1 ORANGE
- ➡ 3 HARD PEARS
- ➡ 3 APPLES

CEREBRAL ENERGY

Once you're living a healthy lifestyle eating mainly macro nutrient foods, this juice will help give your brain that energy to get you through that rough day you have coming.

- ➡ 1 ORANGE
- ➡ 1 HARD PEAR
- ➡ 1 YAM
- ➡ 1 GRAPEFRUIT
- ➡ 1 APPLE

THE FENNEL CLUB

This juice is good for headaches, migraines, and believe it or not, helps with night blindness!

- ➡ 1 FENNEL BULB
- ➡ 1/2 BEET WITH GREENS
- ➡ 2 APPLES

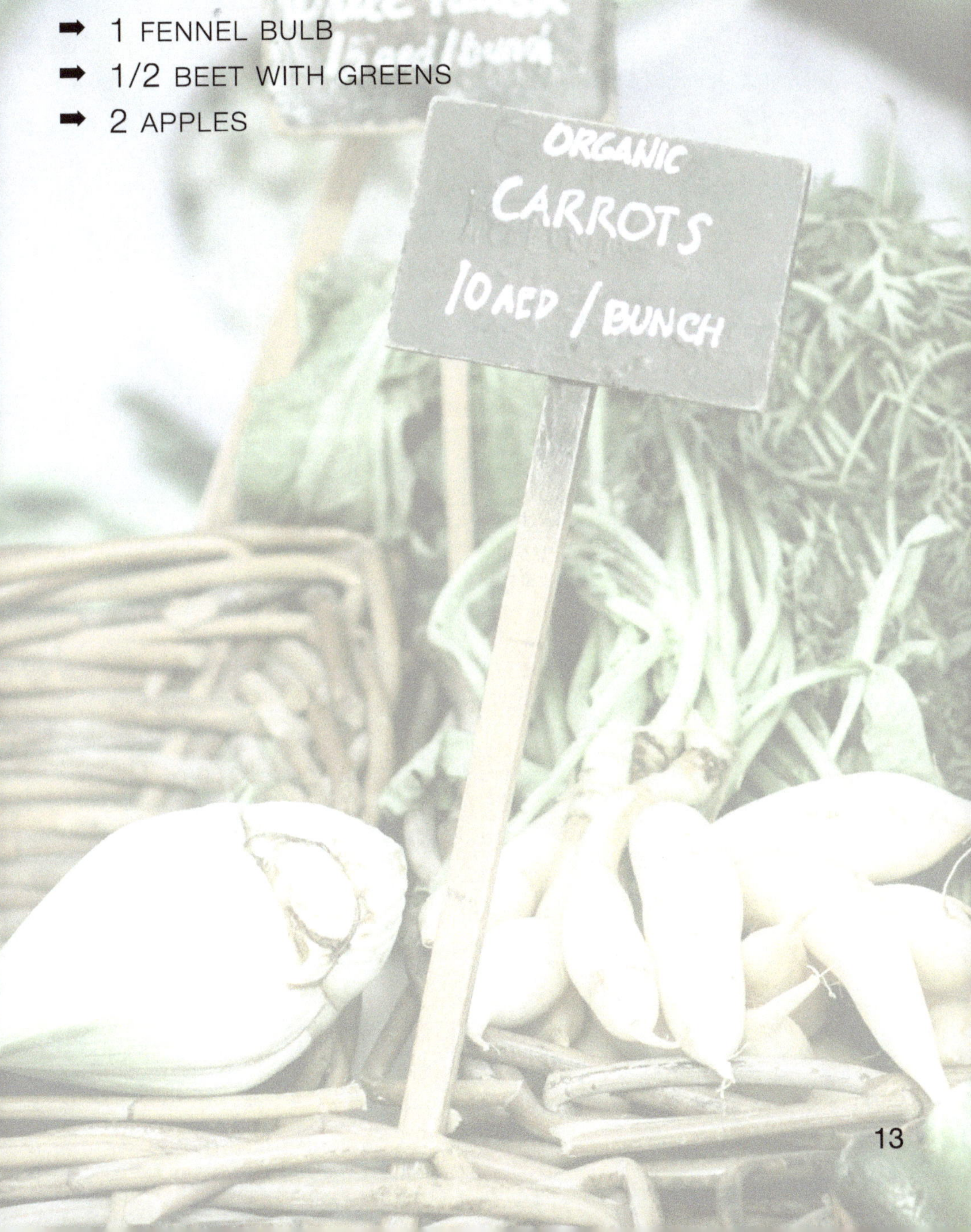

BACTERIA KILLER

Garlic has been known to help with blood clotting, reducing blood pressure, lowering bad cholesterol, and many other good things. Not only does it boost your immune system, it's been known to help in the recovery of those who have had heart attacks. So many benefits that haven't even been mentioned here make it a worthwhile drink to annoy your friends with.

➡ 2 TOMATOES
➡ 2 APPLES
➡ 1 CLOVE OF GARLIC
➡ SPRIG OF PARSLEY

THE CANCER KILLER

There's a story behind this drink. This mixture of fruits and vegetables was first introduced by Rudolf Breuss. He combined this drink with a tea composed of nettle, marigold, artemisi, monarda, and St. John's Wort over a 42 day period. This combination is said to starve out the cancer. In his thirty years of practice, Mr. Breuss has reported over a 96% success rate attested by over 20,000 patients. Mr. Breuss reached 93 years of age before passing.

- ➡ 1 BEET
- ➡ 1 CARROT
- ➡ 1 STALK CELERY
- ➡ 1/2 POTATO
- ➡ 1 RADISH

Please note that I'm not advocating or confirming that this will actually kill cancer. All I can do is tell you what I've seen work in my life. This was the primary juice my mom drank during her juice fast while on chemo. After that, everything changed and now she's her Oncologist's favorite patient.

Bladder Reliever

Cranberry juice is known to be a powerful healer. For men it helps reduce the risk of prostate cancer and for women it helps defend against yeast infections and urinary tract infections.

- 2 APPLES
- 1-1/4 CUPS OF CRANBERRIES

Watery Cleanse

When you juice the watermelon, you must include the rind. Reason being is that the rind has Vitamin A, zinc, iodine, chlorophyll, and enzymes that help your digestion. This juice will give your kidneys a makeover and make you feel young and energetic again. You can actually add other fruits and vegetables to this drink so feel free to experiment.

➡ 1 WEDGE WATERMELON
➡ 1/2 LB. RED GRAPES

THE AC INFUSER

By AC I don't mean "Air Conditioner" but Vitamin A and C! Great in taste, this drink has 15k I.U. of vitamin A and lots of natural vitamin C. Have anxiety? This drink contains myo-inositol that helps with anxiety and insomnia. This also includes other ingredients that help with digestion. Cantaloupe is very low in calories but full of nutrients which is great for those trying to lose weight.

- ➡ 1 CANTALOUPE
- ➡ 5 ICE CUBES
- ➡ 2 TBS. OF SUCANAT
- ➡ DASH OF CINNAMON

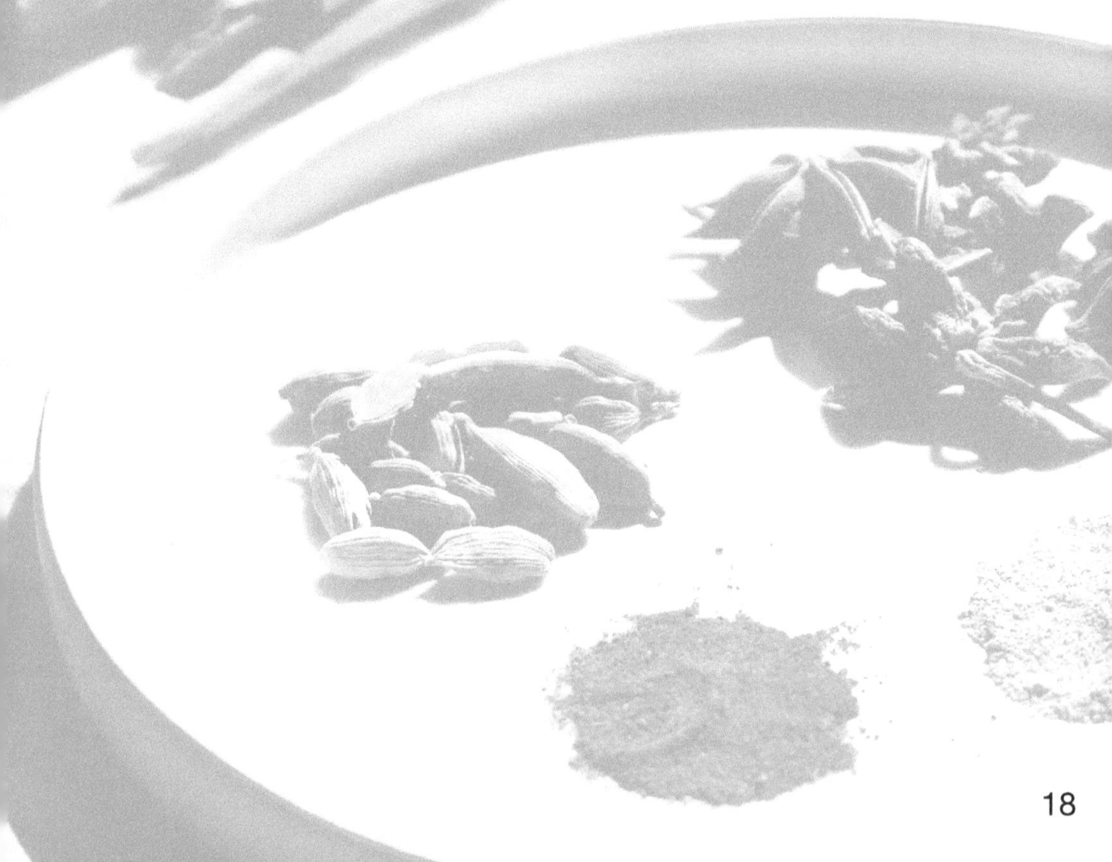

Teas

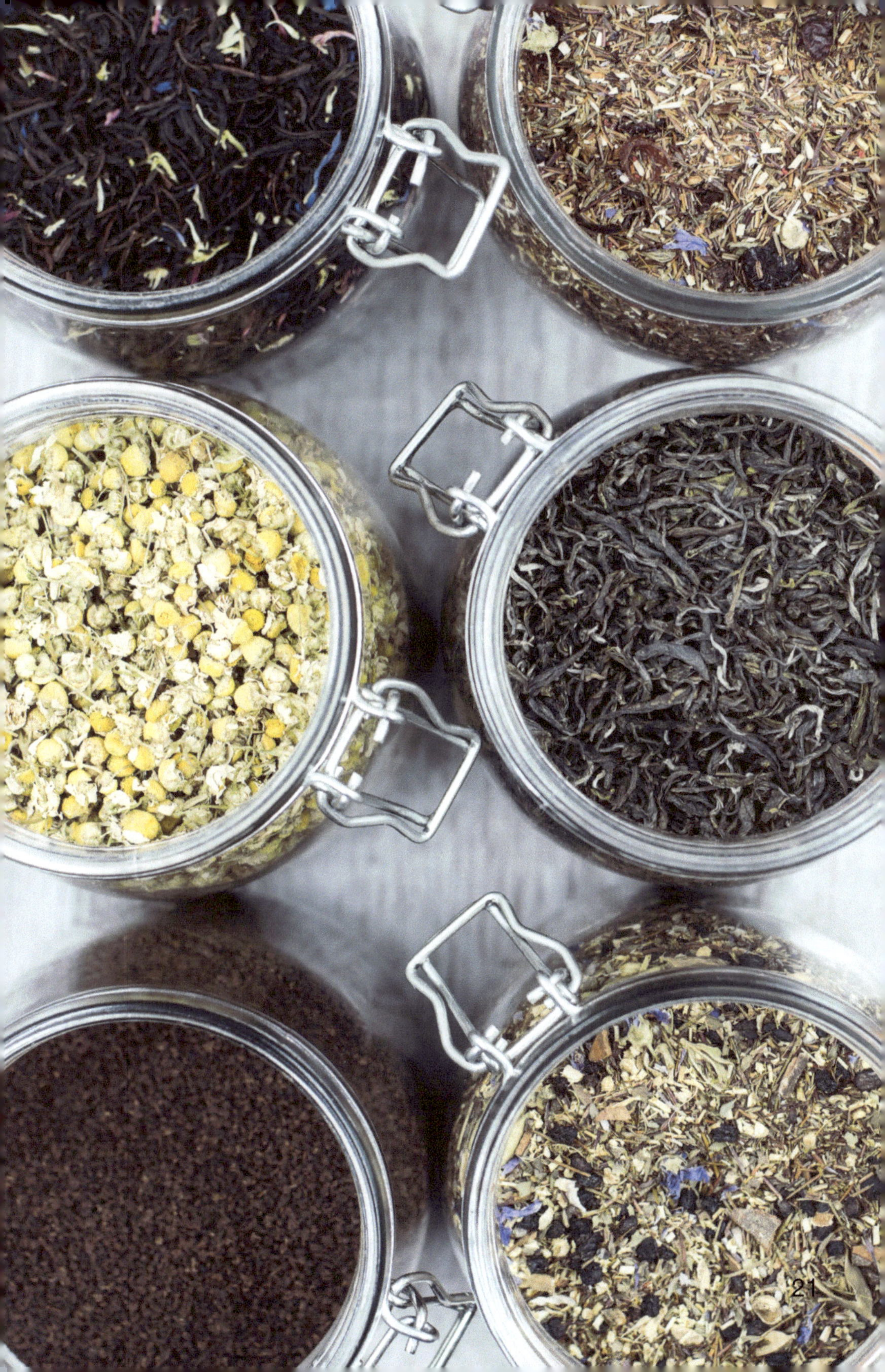

Introduction to Teas

Teas have a way of helping us in life. From digestion, to managing stress, to allergies… The following teas are something that my wife and I use all the time.

Chamomile

Chamomile tea is soothing to the stomach. It's also been used to treat several digestive ailments such as nausea and gas.

Lavender

Lavender tea is helpful with anxiety, stress, and insomnia. It can also aid in depression and has been known to help reduce pain.

Nettle

Nettle tea is known to be high in nutrients, including vitamins A, B1, B2, B3, B5, C, iron, magnesium, among many others. I personally use this for helping with my allergies. It's known to help with sneezing, congestion, itching, and inflammation.

Other Teas

There are many other teas out there. I recommend you go out there and start looking into drinking these as a part of your daily routine, but remember, do your due diligence.

Conclusion

Feel free to come up with your own juice recipes!

Keep in mind that certain fruits/vegetables are better than others. That's why this book has pre-made recipes to get you started.

These above were researched by people and have been known to greatly help you on your fasting or your daily regiment.

If you're looking for good documentaries to help you on your own journey, I recommend these:

Fat, Sick, and Nearly Dead - Joe Cross

Fat, Sick, and Nearly Dead 2 - Joe Cross

Super Juice Me! - Jason Vale

Enjoy!

Image Credits

Page 13
Photo by Kate Trysh
https://unsplash.com/photos/s8u1Gv2uF3o

Page 14
Photo by Bryam Blanco
https://unsplash.com/photos/TgpYelSh7zs

Page 15
Photo by engin akyurt
https://unsplash.com/photos/Y5n8mCpvlZU

Page 16
Photo by Anastasia Zhenina
https://unsplash.com/photos/5vAYNUzBMk4

Page 17
Photo by Filip Baotić
https://unsplash.com/photos/X2W6lfhnxK4

Page 18
Photo by Jocelyn Morales
https://unsplash.com/photos/1cxNdPamDoc

Pages 21, 22
Photo by Alice Pasqual
https://unsplash.com/photos/2yZxFxn1938

Page 23
Photo by Mariana Medvedeva
https://unsplash.com/photos/usflE5Yc7PY

Page 24
Photo by Nicolas Ladino Silva
https://unsplash.com/photos/o2DVsV2PnHE

Page 25
Photo by Diego PH
https://unsplash.com/photos/cEAm7FvwgSM